DR. BARBARA MUCUS CLEANSE

Essential guide to full-body cleanse and detox, liver, kidney, lungs, skin, through approved holistic mucus cleanse strategies for optimal health

Ben Hans

Table of Contents

COPYRIGHT © 2023

CHAPTER ONE

Introduction to Mucus and Its Impact on Health

Mucus is a viscous, gel-like substance produced by mucous membranes in the body. While often associated with discomfort and annoyance when dealing with congestion or a runny nose, mucus plays a vital role in maintaining overall health. This article aims to provide a comprehensive exploration of mucus, its functions, composition, production, and its significant impact on health.

Understanding Mucus:

Mucus is a secretion produced by specialized epithelial cells found in various parts of the body, including the respiratory tract, gastrointestinal tract, reproductive organs, and the eyes. It serves as a protective barrier against pathogens, irritants, and foreign particles, preventing them from entering the body's tissues and causing harm. The consistency and composition of mucus vary depending on its location and function within the body.

Composition of Mucus:

Mucus primarily consists of water, glycoproteins known as mucins, electrolytes, antibodies, enzymes, and cellular debris. Mucins, the main component of mucus, give it its characteristic viscosity and adhesive properties. These large, glycosylated proteins form a network that traps foreign particles and microorganisms, facilitating their removal from the body.

Functions of Mucus:

The functions of mucus are diverse and essential for maintaining health:

1. **Protection:** Mucus acts as a physical barrier, trapping pathogens, allergens, and other harmful substances before they can penetrate deeper into the body's tissues. It also contains antimicrobial peptides and antibodies that help neutralize and eliminate pathogens.

2. **Moisturization:** In the respiratory tract, mucus helps keep the airways moist, preventing them from drying out and becoming irritated. This is crucial for maintaining proper lung function and preventing conditions such as bronchitis and asthma.

3. **Ciliary Clearance:** In the respiratory tract, mucus works in conjunction with cilia, tiny hair-like structures lining the airways, to remove trapped particles and microorganisms. Cilia beat in a coordinated manner, propelling mucus and its contents upward toward the throat, where they can be swallowed or expelled through coughing.

4. **Digestion:** In the gastrointestinal tract, mucus lubricates the passage of food, protecting the delicate lining of the

stomach and intestines from damage by gastric acid and digestive enzymes. It also contains enzymes that aid in the breakdown of food molecules for absorption.

5. **Reproductive Health:** Mucus plays a crucial role in fertility and reproduction by providing lubrication and creating a hospitable environment for sperm to travel through the female reproductive tract.

Production of Mucus:

Mucus production is regulated by various factors, including hormonal signals, neural input, and inflammatory mediators. Goblet cells, found in the epithelial lining of mucous membranes, are responsible for synthesizing and secreting mucins and other components of mucus. The production and secretion of mucus are tightly regulated to maintain a balance between protection and obstruction.

Impact of Mucus on Health:

While mucus is essential for health, its overproduction or abnormal composition can contribute to various medical conditions:

1. **Respiratory Conditions:** Excessive mucus production or impaired clearance can lead to respiratory symptoms such as congestion, coughing, and difficulty breathing. Conditions like chronic bronchitis, cystic fibrosis, and asthma are

characterized by abnormal mucus production and clearance mechanisms.

2. **Gastrointestinal Disorders:** Alterations in mucus production or quality can contribute to gastrointestinal disorders such as inflammatory bowel disease (IBD), gastritis, and peptic ulcers. In IBD, for example, abnormalities in the mucus layer lining the intestines can compromise barrier function and increase susceptibility to inflammation and tissue damage.

3. **Reproductive Issues:** Abnormalities in cervical mucus production can affect fertility by impairing sperm motility or hindering their ability to reach and fertilize the egg. Conditions such as cervical dysplasia or cervical mucus hostility can interfere with conception and increase the risk of infertility.

4. **Infections:** Mucus provides a favorable environment for the growth and survival of pathogens, making it a common site of infection. Respiratory viruses such as influenza and rhinovirus often target the respiratory tract's mucus membranes, leading to symptoms of the common cold or flu.

Conclusion:

In conclusion, mucus is a multifunctional substance essential for maintaining health and protecting the body from harm. Its diverse roles in protection, lubrication, and immune defense highlight its significance in various physiological processes. However, disruptions in mucus production or composition can contribute to the development of several medical conditions affecting the respiratory, gastrointestinal, and reproductive systems. Further research into the regulation of mucus production and its role in health and disease is essential for developing targeted therapeutic interventions to address mucus-related disorders.

CHAPTER TWO

Understanding the Role of Herbal Remedies in Mucus Cleansing

Herbal remedies have been used for centuries in traditional medicine systems worldwide to address various health concerns, including respiratory issues associated with excessive mucus production. These remedies often include a variety of plant-based ingredients known for their expectorant, mucolytic, and anti-inflammatory properties. This article aims to explore the role of herbal remedies in mucus cleansing, focusing on their mechanisms of action, popular herbs used, and their effectiveness in promoting respiratory health.

Mechanisms of Action:

Herbal remedies for mucus cleansing exert their effects through several mechanisms:

1. **Expectorant Action:** Many herbs possess expectorant properties, meaning they promote the expulsion of mucus from the respiratory tract by thinning and loosening it. This action helps alleviate congestion and facilitates the clearance of mucus from the airways, making it easier to breathe.

2. **Mucolytic Activity:** Some herbs contain compounds that directly break down mucus, making it less viscous and easier to expel. These mucolytic agents help reduce the thickness

of mucus, promoting its clearance and relieving respiratory symptoms.

3. **Anti-inflammatory Effects:** Chronic inflammation of the respiratory tract can contribute to excessive mucus production and congestion. Certain herbs possess anti-inflammatory properties that help reduce inflammation in the airways, alleviating swelling and discomfort associated with respiratory conditions.

4. **Antimicrobial Action:** In addition to promoting mucus clearance, some herbal remedies exhibit antimicrobial activity, helping to combat respiratory infections caused by bacteria, viruses, or fungi. By targeting pathogens directly, these herbs can aid in resolving infections and preventing their recurrence.

Popular Herbs Used in Mucus Cleansing:

Several herbs are commonly used in herbal remedies for mucus cleansing and respiratory health. Some of the most popular include:

1. **Eucalyptus (Eucalyptus globulus):** Eucalyptus contains cineole, a compound known for its expectorant and decongestant properties. Inhalation of eucalyptus vapors or consumption of eucalyptus tea can help loosen mucus and relieve respiratory congestion.

2. **Peppermint (Mentha piperita):** Peppermint contains menthol, which acts as a natural decongestant and bronchodilator, helping to open up the airways and ease breathing. Peppermint tea or steam inhalation with peppermint oil can help alleviate respiratory symptoms.

3. **Ginger (Zingiber officinale):** Ginger has anti-inflammatory and mucolytic properties, making it useful for reducing inflammation in the respiratory tract and promoting mucus clearance. Ginger tea or fresh ginger added to meals can help soothe respiratory discomfort.

4. **Licorice (Glycyrrhiza glabra):** Licorice root contains glycyrrhizin, a compound with expectorant and anti-inflammatory effects. Licorice tea or supplements may help reduce mucus production and alleviate coughing associated with respiratory conditions.

5. **Thyme (Thymus vulgaris):** Thyme contains thymol, a compound with antimicrobial properties that can help fight respiratory infections. Thyme tea or steam inhalation with thyme oil can help relieve congestion and support respiratory health.

Effectiveness of Herbal Remedies:

While herbal remedies have been used for generations to promote mucus cleansing and respiratory health, their effectiveness varies depending on the specific herbs used, individual responses, and the underlying cause of respiratory symptoms. Clinical studies investigating the efficacy of herbal remedies for mucus cleansing have yielded mixed results, with some demonstrating beneficial effects, while others show inconclusive evidence.

However, many people report subjective improvements in respiratory symptoms after using herbal remedies, suggesting that they may offer symptomatic relief for conditions such as cough, congestion, and bronchitis. Additionally, herbal remedies are generally considered safe when used appropriately, with fewer adverse effects compared to conventional medications.

Conclusion:

Herbal remedies play a valuable role in promoting mucus cleansing and supporting respiratory health through their expectorant, mucolytic, anti-inflammatory, and antimicrobial properties. While scientific evidence supporting their effectiveness is limited and further research is needed, many individuals find relief from respiratory symptoms by incorporating herbal remedies into their wellness routines. As with any natural remedy, it's essential to consult with a healthcare professional before using herbal supplements, especially if you have underlying health conditions or are taking medications.

CHAPTER THREE

Identifying Common Culprits: Foods That Contribute to Excess Mucus

Excessive mucus production can lead to discomfort and respiratory symptoms such as congestion, coughing, and throat irritation. While mucus plays a vital role in protecting the body from pathogens and irritants, certain foods can exacerbate mucus production or promote its thickening, contributing to respiratory issues. This article aims to explore common culprits among foods that may contribute to excess mucus production and exacerbate respiratory symptoms.

Dairy Products:

Dairy products, including milk, cheese, yogurt, and ice cream, are often cited as potential contributors to increased mucus production. While the evidence supporting this claim is mixed, some individuals report experiencing heightened mucus production or congestion after consuming dairy. The exact mechanism behind this phenomenon is not fully understood but may be related to the presence of certain proteins or fats in dairy products that can stimulate mucus secretion.

Processed Foods:

Processed foods high in refined sugars, unhealthy fats, and artificial additives may promote inflammation in the body, including the respiratory tract. This inflammation can trigger an immune response, leading to increased mucus production as the body attempts to protect itself from perceived threats. Additionally, processed foods are often low in fiber and essential nutrients, which are important for maintaining optimal respiratory health.

Sugary Foods and Beverages:

High-sugar foods and beverages, such as sodas, candies, pastries, and sweetened snacks, can exacerbate mucus production and inflammation in the body. Consuming excessive amounts of sugar can disrupt immune function and promote the growth of harmful bacteria and yeast in the gut, potentially leading to respiratory issues. Furthermore, sugary foods can spike blood sugar levels, leading to fluctuations in energy levels and increased susceptibility to infections.

Fried and Fatty Foods:

Fried and fatty foods, such as deep-fried snacks, fast food, and fatty meats, are high in unhealthy fats that can promote inflammation and mucus production in the body. These foods are often low in fiber and antioxidants, which are important for supporting immune function and reducing inflammation. Consuming large amounts of fried and fatty foods may exacerbate respiratory symptoms and contribute to chronic conditions such as asthma and bronchitis.

Gluten-containing Foods:

Some individuals with gluten sensitivity or celiac disease may experience increased mucus production or respiratory symptoms after consuming gluten-containing foods such as wheat, barley, and rye. While the exact mechanism is not fully understood, it is believed that gluten consumption may trigger an inflammatory response in susceptible individuals, leading to respiratory discomfort and congestion.

Alcohol and Caffeine:

Alcohol and caffeine are known to have dehydrating effects on the body, which can thicken mucus and exacerbate respiratory symptoms such as coughing and throat irritation. Additionally, alcoholic beverages and caffeinated drinks such as coffee and tea may irritate the respiratory tract and promote inflammation, further contributing to mucus production and discomfort.

Conclusion:

While the relationship between diet and mucus production is complex and varies among individuals, certain foods may contribute to excess mucus production and exacerbate respiratory symptoms in susceptible individuals. Dairy products, processed foods, sugary foods and beverages, fried and fatty foods, gluten-containing foods, alcohol, and caffeine are among the common culprits that may worsen respiratory issues.

However, it's essential to note that individual responses to these foods can vary, and not everyone will experience adverse effects. Maintaining a balanced diet rich in fruits, vegetables, whole grains, lean proteins, and healthy fats is key to supporting optimal respiratory health and minimizing mucus-related discomfort. If you suspect that certain foods may be exacerbating your respiratory symptoms, consider keeping a food diary and consulting with a healthcare professional or registered dietitian for personalized dietary guidance.

CHAPTER FOUR

The Science Behind Herbal Ingredients: How They Work to Clear Mucus

Herbal ingredients have been utilized for centuries in traditional medicine systems across cultures to address various health concerns, including respiratory issues associated with excessive mucus production. These herbs contain bioactive compounds with expectorant, mucolytic, anti-inflammatory, and antimicrobial properties, which play a crucial role in clearing mucus from the respiratory tract. This article aims to delve into the scientific mechanisms underlying the effectiveness of herbal ingredients in clearing mucus and promoting respiratory health.

Expectorant Action:

Many herbs exert expectorant effects, meaning they facilitate the expulsion of mucus from the respiratory tract by increasing the volume or hydration of respiratory secretions. This action helps alleviate congestion and promotes the clearance of mucus, making it easier to breathe. One of the primary mechanisms by which herbs exert expectorant effects is by stimulating the secretion of respiratory fluids, including mucus, from the mucous glands in the airway epithelium. Additionally, certain herbs may enhance the coordination of ciliary movement in the respiratory tract, aiding in the removal of mucus and trapped particles.

Mucolytic Activity:

Some herbs contain bioactive compounds with mucolytic properties, meaning they help break down and liquefy thick mucus, making it easier to expel from the airways. These compounds work by disrupting the molecular structure of mucus, reducing its viscosity and adhesiveness. One well-known mucolytic compound found in certain herbs is N-acetylcysteine (NAC), which acts by cleaving disulfide bonds within mucin proteins, thereby reducing mucus viscosity and promoting its clearance. Other herbs may contain enzymes or surfactants that facilitate the breakdown and dispersion of mucus in the respiratory tract.

Anti-inflammatory Effects:

Chronic inflammation of the respiratory tract can contribute to excessive mucus production and respiratory symptoms such as congestion and coughing. Many herbs possess anti-inflammatory properties that help reduce inflammation in the airways, alleviating swelling and discomfort associated with respiratory conditions. These herbs may inhibit the production or activity of pro-inflammatory mediators, such as cytokines and leukotrienes, thereby dampening the inflammatory response in the respiratory tract. By reducing inflammation, these herbs help restore normal mucous membrane function and promote mucus clearance.

Antimicrobial Action:

In addition to promoting mucus clearance, some herbs exhibit antimicrobial activity, helping to combat respiratory infections caused by bacteria, viruses, or fungi. These herbs may contain compounds with broad-spectrum antimicrobial properties, including phenolic compounds, flavonoids, and alkaloids. By targeting pathogens directly, these herbs help prevent the proliferation of microorganisms in the respiratory tract, thereby reducing the burden of infection and promoting recovery. Additionally, certain herbs may enhance immune function, supporting the body's natural defense mechanisms against respiratory infections.

Conclusion:

Herbal ingredients offer a rich source of bioactive compounds with expectorant, mucolytic, anti-inflammatory, and antimicrobial properties, which play a crucial role in clearing mucus and promoting respiratory health. Through their diverse mechanisms of action, these herbs help alleviate congestion, reduce inflammation, combat respiratory infections, and facilitate the removal of mucus from the airways. While further research is needed to elucidate the specific mechanisms of individual herbs and their efficacy in treating respiratory conditions, the scientific evidence supporting the use of herbal ingredients for mucus clearance is promising. Incorporating herbal remedies into respiratory care regimens may offer a natural and effective approach to managing mucus-related respiratory symptoms.

CHAPTER FIVE

Preparing Your Body for a Mucus Cleanse: Diet and Lifestyle Changes

Before embarking on a mucus cleanse, it's essential to prepare your body by making dietary and lifestyle changes that support respiratory health and promote mucus clearance. This preparatory phase aims to optimize your body's natural detoxification mechanisms, enhance immune function, and minimize factors that contribute to excess mucus production. In this article, we'll explore key diet and lifestyle adjustments to consider before starting a mucus cleanse.

1. Hydration:

Proper hydration is essential for maintaining optimal respiratory health and promoting mucus clearance. Drinking an adequate amount of water helps keep respiratory secretions thin and facilitates their removal from the airways. Aim to drink at least eight glasses of water per day, and consider incorporating hydrating beverages such as herbal teas, broths, and fresh fruit juices into your daily routine.

2. Anti-Inflammatory Diet:

Following an anti-inflammatory diet can help reduce inflammation in the respiratory tract and minimize mucus production. Focus on consuming whole, nutrient-dense foods rich in antioxidants, such as fruits, vegetables, whole grains, legumes, nuts, and seeds. Limit or avoid processed foods, refined sugars, unhealthy fats, and artificial additives, which can promote inflammation and exacerbate respiratory symptoms.

3. Elimination of Mucus-Forming Foods:

Certain foods may contribute to excess mucus production or promote its thickening in the respiratory tract. Consider temporarily eliminating or reducing consumption of dairy products, processed foods, sugary foods and beverages, fried and fatty foods, gluten-containing foods, alcohol, and caffeine. Pay attention to how your body responds to these dietary changes and adjust accordingly.

4. Herbal Support:

Incorporating herbs with expectorant, mucolytic, and anti-inflammatory properties into your diet can help prepare your body for a mucus cleanse. Consider adding herbs such as ginger, turmeric, peppermint, eucalyptus, licorice root, and thyme to your meals or enjoying them as teas. These herbs can help thin mucus, reduce inflammation, and support respiratory health.

5. Steam Therapy:

Steam therapy is a natural method for loosening mucus and clearing congestion from the respiratory tract. Consider incorporating steam inhalation into your daily routine by filling a bowl with hot water, adding a few drops of essential oils such as eucalyptus or peppermint, and inhaling the steam for several minutes. This can help hydrate and soothe the airways, making it easier to expel mucus.

6. Regular Exercise:

Regular physical activity can help improve respiratory function and promote mucus clearance by increasing blood flow and circulation throughout the body. Engage in moderate-intensity exercise such as walking, cycling, swimming, or yoga for at least 30 minutes per day. Be mindful of your breathing during exercise and practice deep breathing techniques to help clear mucus from the airways.

7. Stress Management:

Chronic stress can weaken the immune system and exacerbate inflammation in the body, contributing to respiratory issues. Incorporate stress-reduction techniques such as mindfulness meditation, deep breathing exercises, yoga, tai chi, or progressive muscle relaxation into your daily routine. Prioritize self-care activities that promote relaxation and emotional well-being.

8. Adequate Sleep:

Getting enough quality sleep is essential for supporting immune function, reducing inflammation, and promoting overall health. Aim for 7-9 hours of restful sleep per night, and establish a regular sleep schedule to optimize your body's natural circadian rhythms. Create a relaxing bedtime routine, avoid caffeine and electronic devices before bed, and create a comfortable sleep environment conducive to restorative sleep.

Conclusion:

Preparing your body for a mucus cleanse involves adopting dietary and lifestyle changes that support respiratory health, promote mucus clearance, and enhance overall well-being. By hydrating adequately, following an anti-inflammatory diet, eliminating mucus-forming foods, incorporating herbal support, practicing steam therapy, engaging in regular exercise, managing stress, and prioritizing sleep, you can optimize your body's natural detoxification mechanisms and lay the foundation for a successful mucus cleanse. Be mindful of your body's response to these changes and consult with a healthcare professional if you have any underlying health conditions or concerns.

CHAPTER SIX

Dr. Barbara's Herbal Mucus Cleanse Protocol: Step-by-Step Guide

Dr. Barbara's Herbal Mucus Cleanse Protocol offers a comprehensive approach to clearing excess mucus from the respiratory tract and promoting respiratory health using natural herbal remedies. This step-by-step guide outlines the protocol's key principles and provides practical instructions for implementing it effectively.

Step 1: Preparation Phase

Before starting the herbal mucus cleanse, it's essential to prepare your body by making dietary and lifestyle changes that support respiratory health. Follow these steps during the preparation phase:

1. **Hydration:** Drink plenty of water and hydrating beverages such as herbal teas, broths, and fresh fruit juices to keep respiratory secretions thin and facilitate their removal from the airways.

2. **Anti-Inflammatory Diet:** Follow an anti-inflammatory diet rich in whole, nutrient-dense foods such as fruits, vegetables, whole grains, legumes, nuts, and seeds. Limit or avoid processed foods, refined sugars, unhealthy fats, and artificial additives.

3. **Elimination of Mucus-Forming Foods:** Temporarily eliminate or reduce consumption of dairy products, processed foods, sugary foods and beverages, fried and fatty foods, gluten-containing foods, alcohol, and caffeine, which may contribute to excess mucus production.

4. **Herbal Support:** Incorporate herbs with expectorant, mucolytic, and anti-inflammatory properties into your diet, such as ginger, turmeric, peppermint, eucalyptus, licorice root, and thyme.

5. **Steam Therapy:** Practice steam inhalation with essential oils such as eucalyptus or peppermint to hydrate and soothe the airways, making it easier to expel mucus.

6. **Regular Exercise:** Engage in moderate-intensity exercise such as walking, cycling, swimming, or yoga to improve respiratory function and promote mucus clearance.

7. **Stress Management:** Incorporate stress-reduction techniques such as mindfulness meditation, deep breathing exercises, yoga, tai chi, or progressive muscle relaxation into your daily routine to reduce stress and support immune function.

8. **Adequate Sleep:** Prioritize restful sleep by getting 7-9 hours of quality sleep per night and establishing a regular sleep schedule.

Step 2: Herbal Cleanse Phase

Once you have completed the preparation phase, you are ready to begin the herbal mucus cleanse. Follow these steps to implement the cleanse effectively:

1. **Select Herbal Remedies:** Choose herbal remedies known for their expectorant, mucolytic, and anti-inflammatory properties, such as herbal teas, tinctures, capsules, or extracts. Consult with a qualified herbalist or healthcare professional to determine the most suitable herbs for your individual needs.

2. **Dosage and Administration:** Follow the recommended dosage instructions provided for each herbal remedy, and administer them according to the manufacturer's guidelines. Some herbs may be taken orally as teas, tinctures, or capsules, while others may be used topically or inhaled via steam therapy.

3. **Consistency and Duration:** Consistently take the herbal remedies as directed for the specified duration of the cleanse, which may range from several days to several weeks depending on individual circumstances and severity of symptoms.

4. **Monitor and Adjust:** Pay attention to your body's response to the herbal cleanse and adjust your regimen as needed

based on changes in symptoms, tolerance, or side effects. Consult with a healthcare professional if you experience any adverse reactions or concerns during the cleanse.

5. **Supportive Measures:** Continue to support the cleanse with hydration, a healthy diet, regular exercise, stress management techniques, and adequate sleep to maximize its effectiveness and promote overall well-being.

Step 3: Post-Cleanse Maintenance

After completing the herbal mucus cleanse, transition into a maintenance phase to sustain the benefits and support long-term respiratory health:

1. **Gradual Reintroduction:** Slowly reintroduce eliminated foods back into your diet one at a time and observe how your body responds. Pay attention to any changes in symptoms or mucus production and adjust your diet accordingly.

2. **Continued Herbal Support:** Consider incorporating some of the herbal remedies used during the cleanse into your daily wellness routine to support ongoing respiratory health and mucus clearance.

3. **Lifestyle Modifications:** Maintain healthy lifestyle habits, including hydration, a balanced diet, regular exercise, stress

management, and adequate sleep, to continue supporting respiratory function and overall well-being.

4. **Regular Monitoring:** Monitor your respiratory symptoms and mucus production regularly and seek medical attention if you experience persistent or worsening symptoms that may indicate an underlying health condition.

By following Dr. Barbara's Herbal Mucus Cleanse Protocol step-by-step, you can effectively clear excess mucus from the respiratory tract, promote respiratory health, and support overall well-being using natural herbal remedies. Remember to consult with a qualified healthcare professional or herbalist before starting any new dietary or herbal regimen, especially if you have underlying health conditions or concerns.

CHAPTER SEVEN

Herbal Teas and Infusions for Mucus Reduction

Herbal teas and infusions have been used for centuries as natural remedies to help reduce mucus production, alleviate congestion, and promote respiratory health. These soothing beverages harness the therapeutic properties of various herbs, spices, and botanicals known for their expectorant, mucolytic, anti-inflammatory, and antimicrobial effects. Below are some herbal teas and infusions that can be beneficial for reducing mucus and supporting respiratory function:

1. Peppermint Tea:

- Peppermint contains menthol, which acts as a natural decongestant and can help soothe the respiratory tract.

- Drinking peppermint tea may help alleviate congestion and promote mucus clearance.

2. Ginger Tea:

- Ginger has anti-inflammatory and expectorant properties, making it effective for reducing inflammation in the respiratory tract and thinning mucus.

- Drinking ginger tea can help relieve respiratory symptoms such as coughing and congestion.

3. Eucalyptus Tea:

- Eucalyptus contains cineole, a compound with expectorant and antimicrobial properties.

- Drinking eucalyptus tea or inhaling steam infused with eucalyptus oil can help loosen mucus and ease breathing.

4. Licorice Root Tea:

- Licorice root contains glycyrrhizin, which has expectorant and anti-inflammatory effects.

- Drinking licorice root tea may help reduce mucus production and soothe irritated respiratory tissues.

5. Thyme Tea:

- Thyme contains thymol, a compound with antimicrobial and expectorant properties.

- Drinking thyme tea can help alleviate respiratory infections and promote mucus clearance.

6. Turmeric Tea:

- Turmeric contains curcumin, a compound with potent anti-inflammatory and antioxidant properties.

- Drinking turmeric tea may help reduce inflammation in the respiratory tract and support overall respiratory health.

7. Mullein Tea:

- Mullein is traditionally used as an expectorant and demulcent, helping to expel mucus and soothe irritated respiratory tissues.

- Drinking mullein tea can help alleviate coughing and congestion associated with excessive mucus production.

8. Chamomile Tea:

- Chamomile has anti-inflammatory and soothing properties that can help reduce respiratory discomfort and promote relaxation.

- Drinking chamomile tea may help calm respiratory irritation and support mucus clearance.

9. Oregano Tea:

- Oregano contains carvacrol and thymol, compounds with antimicrobial properties.

- Drinking oregano tea can help combat respiratory infections and promote overall respiratory health.

10. Lemon and Honey Infusion:

- Lemon contains vitamin C, which supports immune function, while honey has antimicrobial and soothing properties.

- Sipping on a warm infusion of lemon and honey can help soothe a sore throat and alleviate respiratory symptoms.

When preparing herbal teas and infusions for mucus reduction, use high-quality organic herbs and botanicals whenever possible. Steep the herbs in hot water for 5-10 minutes to extract their beneficial compounds, and enjoy the warm beverage several times a day as needed to support respiratory health. As always, consult with a healthcare professional before incorporating new herbal remedies into your wellness routine, especially if you have underlying health conditions or are pregnant or breastfeeding.

CHAPTER EIGHT

Incorporating Exercise and Detox Techniques for Enhanced Results

Exercise and detox techniques can complement herbal remedies and dietary changes in promoting mucus reduction and supporting respiratory health. Physical activity helps improve circulation, lymphatic drainage, and overall immune function, while detox techniques aid in eliminating toxins from the body, reducing inflammation, and supporting organ function. Here's how to incorporate exercise and detox techniques for enhanced results in reducing mucus:

1. Aerobic Exercise:

- Engage in aerobic exercises such as brisk walking, jogging, cycling, swimming, or dancing to increase heart rate and improve respiratory function.

- Aerobic exercise helps strengthen the respiratory muscles, enhance lung capacity, and promote mucus clearance through deep breathing and increased circulation.

2. Yoga and Tai Chi:

- Practice gentle, low-impact exercises such as yoga or tai chi to promote relaxation, improve flexibility, and support respiratory health.

- Yoga poses and tai chi movements incorporate deep breathing techniques, which can help clear mucus from the airways and reduce stress-related inflammation.

3. Breathing Exercises:

- Perform specific breathing exercises such as diaphragmatic breathing, pursed lip breathing, or alternate nostril breathing to strengthen respiratory muscles and improve lung function.

- Breathing exercises help increase oxygenation, promote relaxation, and enhance mucus clearance by facilitating deeper inhalation and exhalation.

4. Steam Therapy:

- Incorporate steam therapy into your routine by taking warm showers, sitting in a steam room, or using a humidifier with essential oils such as eucalyptus or peppermint.

- Steam therapy helps hydrate the respiratory tract, loosen mucus, and soothe irritated airways, making it easier to expel mucus and alleviate congestion.

5. Dry Brushing:

- Practice dry brushing before showering to stimulate lymphatic drainage, improve circulation, and remove dead skin cells.

- Dry brushing helps support detoxification by enhancing the body's natural cleansing processes and promoting the elimination of toxins through the skin.

6. Hydrotherapy:

- Take contrast showers or baths by alternating between hot and cold water to stimulate circulation, boost immune function, and support detoxification.

- Hydrotherapy promotes vasodilation and vasoconstriction, which can help improve lymphatic flow and enhance the body's ability to clear toxins.

7. Herbal Detox Teas:

- Drink herbal detox teas containing cleansing herbs such as dandelion root, burdock root, milk thistle, and nettle leaf to support liver function and aid in detoxification.

- Herbal detox teas help eliminate toxins from the body, reduce inflammation, and support overall wellness.

8. Lymphatic Massage:

- Perform gentle lymphatic massage techniques to stimulate lymphatic drainage, reduce fluid retention, and support detoxification.

- Lymphatic massage helps move lymph fluid through the lymphatic system, enhancing the body's ability to remove toxins and waste products.

9. Infrared Sauna:

- Use an infrared sauna to induce sweating, increase circulation, and promote detoxification through the skin.

- Infrared sauna therapy helps eliminate toxins, reduce inflammation, and support immune function, contributing to overall respiratory health.

10. Hydration and Nutrition:

- Stay hydrated by drinking plenty of water throughout the day to support detoxification and maintain optimal hydration levels.

- Eat a nutrient-rich diet high in fruits, vegetables, whole grains, lean proteins, and healthy fats to provide essential vitamins, minerals, and antioxidants that support detoxification and respiratory health.

Incorporating exercise and detox techniques into your routine can enhance the effectiveness of herbal remedies and dietary changes in reducing mucus and supporting respiratory health. Be sure to listen to your body and choose activities that feel comfortable and enjoyable for you. Consult with a healthcare professional before starting any new exercise or detox regimen, especially if you have underlying health conditions or concerns.

CHAPTER NINE

Managing Symptoms and Potential Side Effects During the Cleanse

While a mucus cleanse can offer numerous benefits for respiratory health, it's essential to be mindful of potential symptoms and side effects that may arise during the process. Proper management of these symptoms can help ensure a smoother cleansing experience and optimize the benefits of the cleanse. Here are some strategies for managing symptoms and potential side effects during the cleanse:

1. Increased Mucus Production:

- It's common to experience an initial increase in mucus production during the early stages of a cleanse as the body begins to expel toxins and impurities. This may manifest as nasal congestion, coughing, or throat irritation.

- Stay hydrated by drinking plenty of water and herbal teas to help thin mucus and facilitate its removal from the respiratory tract.

- Use steam therapy or saline nasal rinses to help clear nasal passages and alleviate congestion.

2. Digestive Discomfort:

- Some herbal remedies and dietary changes may cause mild digestive discomfort, such as bloating, gas, or changes in bowel habits, as your body adjusts to the cleanse.

- Eat smaller, more frequent meals to aid digestion and prevent overloading the digestive system.

- Incorporate digestive-supporting herbs such as ginger, fennel, or peppermint into your meals or as herbal teas to alleviate digestive symptoms.

3. Fatigue and Lethargy:

- It's not uncommon to experience temporary fatigue or lethargy during a cleanse, especially during the initial detoxification phase as the body expels toxins and metabolic waste products.

- Prioritize rest and relaxation by getting plenty of sleep and taking breaks throughout the day to recharge.

- Avoid overexertion and engage in gentle exercise such as walking, yoga, or tai chi to promote circulation and energy flow.

4. Headaches and Body Aches:

- Headaches and body aches may occur as a result of toxin release and detoxification processes during the cleanse.

- Stay hydrated to help flush out toxins and maintain electrolyte balance.

- Use gentle massage, stretching, or hot/cold therapy to alleviate muscle tension and promote relaxation.

5. Emotional Release:

- Emotional release is a common phenomenon during detoxification, as stored emotions and stress may be released along with physical toxins.

- Practice mindfulness techniques such as meditation, deep breathing, or journaling to process and release emotions as they arise.

- Seek support from friends, family, or a healthcare professional if you need assistance navigating emotional challenges during the cleanse.

6. Allergic Reactions:

- Some individuals may experience allergic reactions or sensitivities to certain herbs or ingredients used in herbal remedies.

- Monitor your body's response to herbal remedies and discontinue use if you experience any adverse reactions such as itching, swelling, or difficulty breathing.

- Consult with a healthcare professional or herbalist for alternative remedies or recommendations if you have known allergies or sensitivities.

7. Electrolyte Imbalance:

- Increased fluid intake during a cleanse may lead to electrolyte imbalances if not adequately balanced with electrolyte-rich foods or supplements.

- Consume electrolyte-rich foods such as bananas, leafy greens, avocados, and coconut water to maintain electrolyte balance.

- Consider adding a high-quality electrolyte supplement to your regimen if needed, especially if you experience symptoms such as muscle cramps or fatigue.

8. Monitoring Progress:

- Keep track of your symptoms, progress, and overall well-being throughout the cleanse to assess its effectiveness and make any necessary adjustments.

- Listen to your body and honor its needs by adjusting your regimen or seeking additional support as needed.

- Consult with a healthcare professional if you have concerns or experience persistent or severe symptoms during the cleanse.

By proactively managing symptoms and potential side effects during the cleanse, you can optimize your experience and support your body's natural detoxification processes effectively. Remember to be patient and gentle with yourself throughout the process, and prioritize self-care to promote overall well-being. If you have any underlying health conditions or concerns, consult with a healthcare professional before starting any new cleanse or wellness regimen.

CHAPTER TEN

Long-Term Strategies for Maintaining a Mucus-Free Lifestyle

Maintaining a mucus-free lifestyle involves adopting long-term habits and practices that support respiratory health, promote mucus clearance, and minimize factors that contribute to excess mucus production. By incorporating these strategies into your daily routine, you can sustain the benefits of a mucus cleanse and enjoy improved respiratory function and overall well-being over the long term. Here are some long-term strategies for maintaining a mucus-free lifestyle:

1. Balanced Diet:

- Follow a balanced diet rich in fruits, vegetables, whole grains, lean proteins, and healthy fats to provide essential nutrients and antioxidants that support respiratory health.

- Limit or avoid mucus-forming foods such as dairy products, processed foods, sugary foods and beverages, fried and fatty foods, gluten-containing foods, alcohol, and caffeine.

2. Hydration:

- Stay hydrated by drinking plenty of water throughout the day to keep respiratory secretions thin and facilitate their removal from the airways.

- Incorporate hydrating beverages such as herbal teas, broths, and fresh fruit juices into your daily routine.

3. Regular Exercise:

- Engage in regular physical activity to improve respiratory function, promote circulation, and support mucus clearance.

- Include aerobic exercises, strength training, and flexibility exercises in your routine to maintain overall fitness and respiratory health.

4. Stress Management:

- Practice stress-reduction techniques such as mindfulness meditation, deep breathing exercises, yoga, tai chi, or progressive muscle relaxation to reduce stress and promote relaxation.

- Prioritize self-care activities that support emotional well-being and resilience.

5. Healthy Sleep Habits:

- Establish a regular sleep schedule and aim for 7-9 hours of quality sleep per night to support immune function, reduce inflammation, and promote overall well-being.

- Create a relaxing bedtime routine and optimize your sleep environment for restorative sleep.

6. Environmental Factors:

- Minimize exposure to environmental pollutants, allergens, and irritants such as cigarette smoke, air pollution, dust, pet dander, and mold to reduce respiratory symptoms and mucus production.

- Use air purifiers, humidifiers, and proper ventilation to maintain clean indoor air quality and optimize respiratory health.

7. Herbal Support:

- Incorporate herbal remedies with expectorant, mucolytic, and anti-inflammatory properties into your daily routine to support respiratory health.

- Drink herbal teas, use herbal steam inhalations, or take herbal supplements as needed to promote mucus clearance and alleviate respiratory symptoms.

8. Regular Detoxification:

- Implement periodic detoxification protocols such as herbal cleanses, fasting, or dietary resets to support the body's natural detoxification processes and eliminate accumulated toxins.

- Consult with a healthcare professional or holistic practitioner for personalized detoxification recommendations based on your individual needs and health status.

9. Mindful Eating:

- Practice mindful eating by paying attention to your body's hunger and fullness cues, and choosing nourishing foods that support respiratory health.

- Avoid overeating, mindless snacking, or consuming foods that trigger digestive discomfort or inflammation.

10. Ongoing Education and Support:

- Stay informed about the latest research and developments in respiratory health, herbal medicine, and holistic wellness practices.

- Seek support from healthcare professionals, herbalists, or holistic practitioners who can provide guidance, recommendations, and personalized care to support your mucus-free lifestyle journey.

By incorporating these long-term strategies into your lifestyle, you can maintain a mucus-free environment in your respiratory tract, support optimal respiratory function, and promote overall health and well-being. Remember that consistency and commitment to healthy habits are key to long-term success, and be patient with yourself as you navigate your wellness journey. If you have any underlying health conditions or concerns, consult with a healthcare professional for personalized guidance and support.

BONUS: SOME ESSENTIAL HERBAL REMEDIES TO KNOW

Sarsaparilla:

Definition: Sarsaparilla refers to several species of plants belonging to the Smilax genus, including Smilax regelii and Smilax officinalis. It has been used historically in traditional medicine for its potential health benefits, particularly for its purported detoxifying and anti-inflammatory properties.

Ingredients: Sarsaparilla contains various bioactive compounds, including saponins (such as sarsaponin and smilagenin), flavonoids, phenolic acids, and sterols. These compounds are believed to contribute to the herb's medicinal properties, including its potential as a diuretic, blood purifier, and anti-inflammatory agent.

How to Prepare: Sarsaparilla root is typically prepared and consumed as an herbal tea, decoction, or tincture. To make tea, dried sarsaparilla root is steeped in hot water for several minutes before being strained and consumed. Decoctions involve boiling the root in water to extract its active compounds, while tinctures are prepared by steeping the root in alcohol or vinegar.

Dosage: The appropriate dosage of sarsaparilla can vary depending on factors such as age, health status, and the specific preparation being used. It's important to follow the recommended dosage on the product label or consult with a qualified herbalist or healthcare professional for personalized guidance.

How to Use: Sarsaparilla tea or tincture is typically taken orally. It's important to use sarsaparilla products as directed and to discontinue use if any adverse effects occur.

Side Effects: Sarsaparilla is generally considered safe for most people when used in moderate amounts. However, some individuals may experience allergic reactions or digestive upset. It may also interact with certain medications or have adverse effects in individuals with certain health conditions. It's important to use sarsaparilla under the guidance of a healthcare professional and to discontinue use if any adverse effects occur.

Wild Cherry Bark:

Definition: Wild cherry bark, scientifically known as Prunus serotina, is the bark obtained from the black cherry tree native to North America. It has been used traditionally in Native American and folk medicine for its potential health benefits, particularly for respiratory and digestive issues.

Ingredients: Wild cherry bark contains various bioactive compounds, including cyanogenic glycosides (such as prunasin and amygdalin), flavonoids, and phenolic acids. These compounds are believed to contribute to the herb's medicinal properties, including its potential as an expectorant, cough suppressant, and mild sedative.

How to Prepare: Wild cherry bark is typically prepared and consumed as an herbal tea, decoction, or syrup. To make tea, dried wild cherry bark is steeped in hot water for several minutes before being strained and consumed. Decoctions involve boiling the bark in water to extract its active compounds, while syrups are made by simmering the bark with sugar or honey to create a thick, sweet liquid.

Dosage: The appropriate dosage of wild cherry bark can vary depending on factors such as age, health status, and the specific preparation being used. It's important to follow the recommended dosage on the product label or consult with a qualified herbalist or healthcare professional for personalized guidance.

How to Use: Wild cherry bark tea, decoction, or syrup is typically taken orally. It's often consumed to soothe coughs, sore throats, and other respiratory symptoms. It's important to use wild cherry bark products as directed and to discontinue use if any adverse effects occur.

Side Effects: Wild cherry bark is generally considered safe for most people when used in moderate amounts. However, it contains cyanogenic glycosides, which can release cyanide in the body when metabolized. While the risk of cyanide poisoning from consuming wild cherry bark is low when used appropriately, excessive intake or prolonged use may lead to adverse effects. It's important to use wild cherry bark under the guidance of a healthcare professional and to discontinue use if any adverse effects occur.

Yellowdock:

Definition: Yellowdock, scientifically known as Rumex crispus, is a perennial flowering plant native to Europe and western Asia but is also found in North America. It has a long history of use in traditional medicine, particularly among Indigenous peoples, for its potential health benefits.

Ingredients: Yellowdock root contains various bioactive compounds, including anthraquinone glycosides (such as emodin and chrysophanol), tannins, and vitamins (including vitamin A and vitamin C). These compounds are believed to contribute to the herb's medicinal properties, including its potential as a laxative, blood cleanser, and liver tonic.

How to Prepare: Yellowdock root is typically prepared and consumed as an herbal tea, tincture, or capsule. To make tea, dried yellowdock root is steeped in hot water for several minutes before being strained and consumed. Tinctures are prepared by steeping the root in alcohol or vinegar to extract its active compounds.

Dosage: The appropriate dosage of yellowdock can vary depending on factors such as age, health status, and the specific preparation being used. It's important to follow the recommended dosage on the product label or consult with a qualified herbalist or healthcare professional for personalized guidance.

How to Use: Yellowdock tea, tincture, or capsules are typically taken orally. It's often consumed to support digestion, promote bowel regularity, and cleanse the blood. It's important to use yellowdock products as directed and to discontinue use if any adverse effects occur.

Side Effects: Yellowdock is generally considered safe for most people when used in moderate amounts. However, some individuals may experience mild side effects such as gastrointestinal upset or allergic reactions. It may also interact with certain medications or have adverse effects in individuals with certain health conditions. It's important to use yellowdock under the guidance of a healthcare professional and to discontinue use if any adverse effects occur.

Yellowdock Root:

Definition: Yellowdock root, scientifically known as Rumex crispus, is the root of a perennial flowering plant native to Europe and western Asia, also found in North America. It has a long history of use in traditional medicine, particularly among Indigenous peoples, for its potential health benefits.

Ingredients: Yellowdock root contains various bioactive compounds, including anthraquinone glycosides (such as emodin and chrysophanol), tannins, and vitamins (including vitamin A and vitamin C). These compounds are believed to contribute to the herb's medicinal properties, including its potential as a laxative, blood cleanser, and liver tonic.

How to Prepare: Yellowdock root is typically prepared and consumed as an herbal tea, tincture, or capsule. To make tea, dried yellowdock root is steeped in hot water for several minutes before being strained and consumed. Tinctures are prepared by steeping the root in alcohol or vinegar to extract its active compounds.

Dosage: The appropriate dosage of yellowdock root can vary depending on factors such as age, health status, and the specific preparation being used. It's important to follow the recommended dosage on the product label or consult with a qualified herbalist or healthcare professional for personalized guidance.

How to Use: Yellowdock root tea, tincture, or capsules are typically taken orally. It's often consumed to support digestion, promote bowel regularity, and cleanse the blood. It's important to use yellowdock root products as directed and to discontinue use if any adverse effects occur.

Side Effects: Yellowdock root is generally considered safe for most people when used in moderate amounts. However, some individuals may experience mild side effects such as gastrointestinal upset or allergic reactions. It may also interact with certain medications or have adverse effects in individuals with certain health conditions. It's important to use yellowdock root under the guidance of a healthcare professional and to discontinue use if any adverse effects occur.

Agrimony:

Definition: Agrimony, scientifically known as Agrimonia eupatoria, is a perennial herbaceous plant native to Europe, Asia, and North America. It has a long history of use in traditional medicine, particularly in European folk medicine, for its potential health benefits.

Ingredients: Agrimony contains various bioactive compounds, including tannins, flavonoids, phenolic acids, and volatile oils. These compounds are believed to contribute to the herb's medicinal properties, including its potential as an astringent, anti-inflammatory, and digestive aid.

How to Prepare: Agrimony is typically prepared and consumed as an herbal tea, tincture, or poultice. To make tea, dried agrimony leaves and flowers are steeped in hot water for several minutes before being strained and consumed. Tinctures are prepared by steeping the herb in alcohol or vinegar to extract its active compounds.

Dosage: The appropriate dosage of agrimony can vary depending on factors such as age, health status, and the specific preparation being used. It's important to follow the recommended dosage on the product label or consult with a qualified herbalist or healthcare professional for personalized guidance.

How to Use: Agrimony tea, tincture, or poultice is typically taken orally or applied topically. It's often consumed to soothe gastrointestinal issues, such as indigestion and diarrhea, or used externally to treat skin conditions.

Side Effects: Agrimony is generally considered safe for most people when used in moderate amounts. However, some individuals may experience allergic reactions or gastrointestinal upset. It may also interact with certain medications or have adverse effects in individuals with certain health conditions. It's important to use agrimony under the guidance of a healthcare professional and to discontinue use if any adverse effects occur.

Alfalfa:

Definition: Alfalfa, scientifically known as Medicago sativa, is a flowering plant in the pea family native to Asia but cultivated worldwide. It's primarily grown as fodder for livestock, but it has also been used in traditional medicine for its potential health benefits.

Ingredients: Alfalfa contains various bioactive compounds, including vitamins (such as vitamin A, vitamin C, and vitamin K), minerals (including calcium, magnesium, and potassium), amino acids, and phytoestrogens. These compounds are believed to contribute to the herb's medicinal properties, including its potential as a nutritive tonic, diuretic, and hormone balancer.

How to Prepare: Alfalfa is typically consumed as sprouts, herbal tea, or in supplement form (such as capsules or tablets). To make tea, dried alfalfa leaves are steeped in hot water for several minutes before being strained and consumed.

Dosage: The appropriate dosage of alfalfa can vary depending on factors such as age, health status, and the specific preparation being used. It's important to follow the recommended dosage on the product label or consult with a qualified herbalist or healthcare professional for personalized guidance.

How to Use: Alfalfa sprouts, tea, or supplements are typically taken orally. It's often consumed as a dietary supplement to support overall health and well-being, as well as to promote kidney health and hormone balance.

Side Effects: Alfalfa is generally considered safe for most people when consumed in moderate amounts. However, some individuals may experience allergic reactions or digestive upset. It may also interact with certain medications or have adverse effects in individuals with certain health conditions, such as autoimmune diseases or hormone-sensitive conditions. Pregnant or breastfeeding individuals should consult with a healthcare professional before using alfalfa supplements. It's important to use alfalfa under the guidance of a healthcare professional and to discontinue use if any adverse effects occur.

Ashwagandha:

Definition: Ashwagandha, scientifically known as Withaniasomnifera, is a small shrub native to India, the Middle East, and parts of Africa. It has a long history of use in Ayurvedic medicine for its potential health benefits, particularly for its adaptogenic properties.

Ingredients: Ashwagandha root contains various bioactive compounds, including alkaloids (such as withanolides), steroidal lactones, and flavonoids. These compounds are believed to contribute to the herb's medicinal properties, including its potential as an adaptogen, anti-inflammatory, and immune-modulating agent.

How to Prepare: Ashwagandha is typically consumed as a powdered root, herbal tea, tincture, or in supplement form (such as capsules or tablets). To make tea, dried ashwagandha root is steeped in hot water for several minutes before being strained and consumed.

Dosage: The appropriate dosage of ashwagandha can vary depending on factors such as age, health status, and the specific preparation being used. It's important to follow the recommended dosage on the product label or consult with a qualified herbalist or healthcare professional for personalized guidance.

How to Use: Ashwagandha powder, tea, tincture, or supplements are typically taken orally. It's often consumed to support stress management, promote relaxation, and boost overall vitality and well-being.

Side Effects: Ashwagandha is generally considered safe for most people when used in moderate amounts. However, some individuals may experience mild side effects such as gastrointestinal upset or drowsiness. It may also interact with certain medications or have adverse effects in individuals with certain health conditions, such as autoimmune diseases or thyroid disorders. Pregnant or breastfeeding individuals should consult with a healthcare professional before using ashwagandha supplements. It's important to use ashwagandha under the guidance of a healthcare professional and to discontinue use if any adverse effects occur.

Astragalus:

Definition: Astragalus, scientifically known as Astragalus membranaceus, is a flowering plant native to China and Mongolia but also found in other parts of Asia. It has been used for centuries in traditional Chinese medicine for its potential health benefits, particularly for its immune-enhancing properties.

Ingredients: Astragalus root contains various bioactive compounds, including polysaccharides, saponins (such as astragalosides), flavonoids, and amino acids. These compounds are believed to contribute to the herb's medicinal properties, including its potential as an adaptogen, immunomodulator, and anti-inflammatory agent.

How to Prepare: Astragalus is typically consumed as a powdered root, herbal tea, tincture, or in supplement form (such as capsules or tablets). To make tea, dried astragalus root slices are simmered in water for several minutes before being strained and consumed.

Dosage: The appropriate dosage of astragalus can vary depending on factors such as age, health status, and the specific preparation being used. It's important to follow the recommended dosage on the product label or consult with a qualified herbalist or healthcare professional for personalized guidance.

How to Use: Astragalus powder, tea, tincture, or supplements are typically taken orally. It's often consumed to support immune function, promote vitality, and enhance overall well-being.

Side Effects: Astragalus is generally considered safe for most people when used in moderate amounts. However, some individuals may experience mild side effects such as gastrointestinal upset or allergic reactions. It may also interact with certain medications or have adverse effects in individuals with certain health conditions, such as autoimmune diseases or diabetes. Pregnant or breastfeeding individuals should consult with a healthcare professional before using astragalus supplements. It's important to use astragalus under the guidance of a healthcare professional and to discontinue use if any adverse effects occur.

Black Cohosh:

Definition: Black cohosh, scientifically known as Actaea racemosa (formerly Cimicifuga racemosa), is a perennial herb native to North America. It has a long history of use in traditional Native American medicine and later in folk medicine for its potential health benefits, particularly for women's health.

Ingredients: Black cohosh root contains various bioactive compounds, including triterpene glycosides (such as actein and cimicifugoside), phenolic acids, and flavonoids. These compounds are believed to contribute to the herb's medicinal properties, including its potential as a hormone-balancing agent and its ability to relieve menopausal symptoms.

How to Prepare: Black cohosh is typically consumed as a powdered root, herbal tea, tincture, or in supplement form (such as capsules or tablets). To make tea, dried black cohosh root is steeped in hot water for several minutes before being strained and consumed.

Dosage: The appropriate dosage of black cohosh can vary depending on factors such as age, health status, and the specific preparation being used. It's important to follow the recommended dosage on the product label or consult with a qualified herbalist or healthcare professional for personalized guidance.

How to Use: Black cohosh powder, tea, tincture, or supplements are typically taken orally. It's often used by women to support hormonal balance, relieve menopausal symptoms such as hot flashes and night sweats, and promote overall well-being.

Side Effects: Black cohosh is generally considered safe for most people when used in moderate amounts. However, some individuals may experience mild side effects such as gastrointestinal upset or allergic reactions. It may also interact with certain medications or have adverse effects in individuals with certain health conditions, such as liver disease or hormone-sensitive conditions. Pregnant or breastfeeding individuals should consult with a healthcare professional before using black cohosh supplements. It's important to use black cohosh under the guidance of a healthcare professional and to discontinue use if any adverse effects occur.

Blessed Thistle:

Definition: Blessed thistle, scientifically known as Cnicusbenedictus, is an annual or biennial herb native to the Mediterranean region but also found in other parts of Europe, Asia, and North Africa. It has been used historically in traditional medicine for its potential health benefits, particularly for digestive and liver health.

Ingredients: Blessed thistle contains various bioactive compounds, including sesquiterpene lactones (such as cnicin), flavonoids, tannins, and essential oils. These compounds are believed to contribute to the herb's medicinal properties, including its potential as a digestive tonic, appetite stimulant, and liver tonic.

How to Prepare: Blessed thistle is typically consumed as an herbal tea, tincture, or in supplement form (such as capsules or tablets). To make tea, dried blessed thistle leaves and flowers are steeped in hot water for several minutes before being strained and consumed.

Dosage: The appropriate dosage of blessed thistle can vary depending on factors such as age, health status, and the specific preparation being used. It's important to follow the recommended dosage on the product label or consult with a qualified herbalist or healthcare professional for personalized guidance.

How to Use: Blessed thistle tea, tincture, or supplements are typically taken orally. It's often used to support digestion, stimulate appetite, and promote liver health.

Side Effects: Blessed thistle is generally considered safe for most people when used in moderate amounts. However, some individuals may experience mild side effects such as gastrointestinal upset or allergic reactions. It may also interact with certain medications or have adverse effects in individuals with certain health conditions, such as hormone-sensitive conditions or bleeding disorders. Pregnant or breastfeeding individuals should consult with a healthcare professional before using blessed thistle supplements. It's important to use blessed thistle under the guidance of a healthcare professional and to discontinue use if any adverse effects occur.

Cat's Claw:

Definition: Cat's claw, scientifically known as Uncaria tomentosa, is a woody vine native to the Amazon rainforest and other parts of Central and South America. It has been used for centuries in traditional medicine by indigenous peoples for its potential health benefits.

Ingredients: Cat's claw contains various bioactive compounds, including alkaloids (such as oxindole alkaloids and quinovic acid glycosides), polyphenols, and other phytochemicals. These compounds are believed to contribute to the herb's medicinal properties, including its potential as an immune enhancer, anti-inflammatory, and antioxidant.

How to Prepare: Cat's claw is typically consumed as an herbal tea, tincture, or in supplement form (such as capsules or tablets). To make tea, dried cat's claw bark or leaves are steeped in hot water for several minutes before being strained and consumed.

Dosage: The appropriate dosage of cat's claw can vary depending on factors such as age, health status, and the specific preparation being used. It's important to follow the recommended dosage on the product label or consult with a qualified herbalist or healthcare professional for personalized guidance.

How to Use: Cat's claw tea, tincture, or supplements are typically taken orally. It's often used to support immune function, reduce inflammation, and promote overall well-being.

Side Effects: Cat's claw is generally considered safe for most people when used in moderate amounts. However, some individuals may experience mild side effects such as gastrointestinal upset or allergic reactions. It may also interact with certain medications or have adverse effects in individuals with certain health conditions, such as autoimmune diseases or bleeding disorders. Pregnant or breastfeeding individuals should consult with a healthcare professional before using cat's claw supplements. It's important to use cat's claw under the guidance of a healthcare professional and to discontinue use if any adverse effects occur.

Chickweed:

Definition: Chickweed, scientifically known as Stellaria media, is an annual herbaceous plant native to Europe but naturalized in many other parts of the world. It's often considered a common weed but has been used historically in traditional medicine for its potential health benefits.

Ingredients: Chickweed contains various bioactive compounds, including flavonoids, saponins, mucilage, and vitamins (such as vitamin C). These compounds are believed to contribute to the herb's medicinal properties, including its potential as a demulcent, anti-inflammatory, and mild diuretic.

How to Prepare: Chickweed is typically consumed as an herbal tea, infusion, or in fresh salads. To make tea, dried chickweed leaves and flowers are steeped in hot water for several minutes before being strained and consumed. It can also be used topically as a poultice or infused oil for skin conditions.

Dosage: The appropriate dosage of chickweed can vary depending on factors such as age, health status, and the specific preparation being used. It's important to follow the recommended dosage on the product label or consult with a qualified herbalist or healthcare professional for personalized guidance.

How to Use: Chickweed tea, infusion, or fresh leaves are typically taken orally. It's often used to soothe inflammation, support digestion, and promote overall well-being. Topically, chickweed can be applied to the skin to alleviate itching, irritation, or minor wounds.

Side Effects: Chickweed is generally considered safe for most people when consumed in moderate amounts. However, some individuals may experience allergic reactions or gastrointestinal upset. It may also interact with certain medications or have adverse effects in individuals with certain health conditions. Pregnant or breastfeeding individuals should consult with a healthcare professional before using chickweed supplements. It's important to use chickweed under the guidance of a healthcare professional and to discontinue use if any adverse effects occur.

Cleavers:

Definition: Cleavers, scientifically known as Galium aparine, is a herbaceous annual plant native to Europe, North America, Asia, and Australia. It has a long history of use in traditional medicine for its potential health benefits.

Ingredients: Cleavers contains various bioactive compounds, including iridoid glycosides, flavonoids, tannins, and mucilage. These compounds are believed to contribute to the herb's medicinal properties, including its potential as a diuretic, lymphatic tonic, and mild astringent.

How to Prepare: Cleavers is typically consumed as an herbal tea, infusion, or in fresh salads. To make tea, dried cleavers leaves and stems are steeped in hot water for several minutes before being strained and consumed. It can also be used topically as a poultice or infused oil for skin conditions.

Dosage: The appropriate dosage of cleavers can vary depending on factors such as age, health status, and the specific preparation being used. It's important to follow the recommended dosage on the product label or consult with a qualified herbalist or healthcare professional for personalized guidance.

How to Use: Cleavers tea, infusion, or fresh leaves are typically taken orally. It's often used to support lymphatic drainage, promote urinary tract health, and soothe inflammation. Topically, cleavers can be applied to the skin to alleviate itching, irritation, or minor wounds.

Side Effects: Cleavers is generally considered safe for most people when consumed in moderate amounts. However, some individuals may experience allergic reactions or gastrointestinal upset. It may also interact with certain medications or have adverse effects in individuals with certain health conditions. Pregnant or breastfeeding individuals should consult with a healthcare professional before using cleavers supplements. It's important to use cleavers under the guidance of a healthcare professional and to discontinue use if any adverse effects occur.

Eucalyptus:

Definition: Eucalyptus refers to a genus of flowering trees and shrubs, primarily native to Australia but also found in other parts of the world. Eucalyptus essential oil, extracted from the leaves of certain species, has a long history of use in traditional medicine for its potential health benefits.

Ingredients: Eucalyptus essential oil contains various bioactive compounds, including eucalyptol (cineole), terpenes, and flavonoids. These compounds are believed to contribute to the oil's medicinal properties, including its potential as an expectorant, decongestant, antiseptic, and anti-inflammatory.

How to Prepare: Eucalyptus essential oil can be used in aromatherapy, diffused in the air, or diluted and applied topically to the skin. It can also be added to steam inhalations or chest rubs to help relieve respiratory symptoms.

Dosage: The appropriate dosage of eucalyptus essential oil can vary depending on factors such as age, health status, and the specific application being used. It's important to follow the recommended dosage on the product label or consult with a qualified aromatherapist or healthcare professional for personalized guidance.

How to Use: Eucalyptus essential oil can be used aromatically, topically, or internally, depending on the intended application. It's often used to alleviate respiratory congestion, soothe sore muscles, promote relaxation, and support overall well-being.

Side Effects: Eucalyptus essential oil is generally considered safe for most people when used appropriately. However, it can be toxic if ingested in large amounts and should not be applied directly to the skin without proper dilution. Some individuals may experience allergic reactions or respiratory irritation when exposed to eucalyptus oil. It's important to use eucalyptus oil with caution, especially around children and pets. Pregnant or breastfeeding individuals should consult with a healthcare professional before using eucalyptus oil. If any adverse effects occur, discontinue use and seek medical attention.

Blood Purifier:

Definition: Blood purifiers are herbal remedies or dietary supplements believed to cleanse or detoxify the blood, often promoting overall health and well-being. They are thought to support the body's natural detoxification processes and improve blood circulation.

Ingredients: Blood purifiers may contain a variety of herbs and botanical extracts known for their purported cleansing and detoxifying properties. Common ingredients include burdock root, red clover, dandelion root, and yellow dock root, among others.

How to Prepare: Blood purifiers are typically available in various forms, including capsules, tablets, powders, and liquid extracts. They are usually taken orally with water or juice, following the recommended dosage on the product label.

Dosage: The dosage of blood purifiers can vary depending on the specific product and individual needs. It's important to adhere to the recommended dosage on the product label or consult with a healthcare professional for personalized guidance.

How to Use: Blood purifiers are typically taken orally, either with water or mixed into beverages. They are often used as part of a detoxification regimen or to support overall health and vitality.

Side Effects: While blood purifiers are generally considered safe for most people when used as directed, some individuals may experience side effects such as digestive discomfort, allergic reactions, or interactions with medications. It's important to consult with a healthcare provider before starting any new supplement regimen, especially if you have underlying health conditions or are taking medications.

Blue Vervain:

Definition: Blue vervain, also known as Verbena hastata, is a perennial herb native to North America. It has been used in traditional medicine for centuries to treat various ailments, including anxiety, insomnia, and digestive issues.

Ingredients: Blue vervain contains several active compounds, including aucubin, verbenalin, and volatile oils. These compounds are believed to contribute to the herb's medicinal properties.

How to Prepare: Blue vervain is typically consumed as a tea or tincture. To make tea, dried blue vervain leaves and flowers are steeped in hot water for several minutes before being strained and consumed. Tinctures are prepared by steeping the herb in alcohol or vinegar to extract its active compounds.

Dosage: The appropriate dosage of blue vervain can vary depending on factors such as age, health status, and the specific preparation being used. It's important to follow the recommended dosage on the product label or consult with a qualified herbalist or healthcare professional for personalized guidance.

How to Use: Blue vervain tea or tincture is typically taken orally. It can be consumed on its own or mixed with honey or other herbal teas for added flavor.

Side Effects: While blue vervain is generally considered safe for most people when used in moderation, excessive intake may cause digestive upset or allergic reactions in some individuals. Pregnant or breastfeeding women should avoid blue vervain due to its potential to stimulate uterine contractions. As with any herbal remedy, it's important to consult with a healthcare provider before using blue vervain, especially if you have underlying health conditions or are taking medications.

Bio Ferro Tonic:

Definition: Bio Ferro Tonic is a dietary supplement primarily composed of herbs and minerals. It's often marketed as a natural way to support overall health, particularly by promoting blood health and circulation.

Ingredients: Typical ingredients in Bio Ferro Tonic may include a blend of herbs such as burdock root, yellow dock root, sarsaparilla root, and cascara sagrada bark, along with minerals like iron and potassium phosphate.

How to Prepare: Bio Ferro Tonic usually comes in liquid form and is typically taken orally. It's important to follow the instructions on the product label for dosage and administration.

Dosage: The dosage can vary depending on the specific product and individual needs. It's crucial to consult with a healthcare professional or follow the recommended dosage on the product label to avoid potential side effects.

How to Use: Bio Ferro Tonic is often taken by adding the recommended dosage to water or juice and consuming it orally. It's important to shake the bottle well before use and store it according to the manufacturer's instructions.

Side Effects: While Bio Ferro Tonic is generally considered safe when used as directed, some individuals may experience side effects such as digestive discomfort, allergic reactions, or interactions with medications. It's essential to consult with a healthcare provider before starting any new supplement regimen, especially if you have underlying health conditions or are taking medications.

Bladderwrack:

Definition: Bladderwrack is a type of seaweed or marine algae commonly used in traditional medicine and as a dietary supplement. It's known for its potential health benefits, particularly related to thyroid health and weight management.

Ingredients: Bladderwrack contains various nutrients, including iodine, vitamins, minerals, and antioxidants. The primary active components are iodine and fucoidan, a type of carbohydrate found in brown seaweeds.

How to Prepare: Bladderwrack supplements are available in various forms, including capsules, powders, and liquid extracts. They can be taken orally with water or added to smoothies and other beverages.

Dosage: The appropriate dosage of bladderwrack can vary based on factors such as age, health status, and the specific product being used. It's essential to follow the recommended dosage on the product label or consult with a healthcare professional for personalized guidance.

How to Use: Bladderwrack supplements are typically taken orally, either with water or mixed into food or beverages. It's important to follow the instructions on the product label and avoid exceeding the recommended dosage.

Side Effects: While bladderwrack is generally considered safe for most people when used in moderation, excessive intake of iodine from bladderwrack supplements can cause thyroid dysfunction and other adverse effects. Individuals with thyroid disorders, iodine sensitivity, or certain medical conditions should exercise caution and consult with a healthcare provider before using bladderwrack supplements. Common side effects may include digestive upset, allergic reactions, or interactions with medications.

Ginseng:

Definition: Ginseng refers to several species of perennial plants belonging to the Panax genus, including Panax ginseng (Asian ginseng) and Panax quinquefolius (American ginseng). Ginseng has been used for centuries in traditional medicine, particularly in East Asia, for its potential health benefits.

Ingredients: Ginseng root contains various bioactive compounds, including ginsenosides, polysaccharides, and peptides. These compounds are believed to contribute to the herb's medicinal properties, including its potential as an adaptogen, immune enhancer, and cognitive booster.

How to Prepare: Ginseng is typically consumed as a powdered root, herbal tea, tincture, or in supplement form (such as capsules or tablets). To make tea, dried ginseng root slices are simmered in water for several minutes before being strained and consumed.

Dosage: The appropriate dosage of ginseng can vary depending on factors such as age, health status, and the specific preparation being used. It's important to follow the recommended dosage on the product label or consult with a qualified herbalist or healthcare professional for personalized guidance.

How to Use: Ginseng powder, tea, tincture, or supplements are typically taken orally. It's often used to support energy levels, enhance cognitive function, and promote overall well-being.

Side Effects: Ginseng is generally considered safe for most people when used in moderate amounts. However, some individuals may experience mild side effects such as insomnia, gastrointestinal upset, or headaches. It may also interact with certain medications or have adverse effects in individuals with certain health conditions, such as high blood pressure or diabetes. Pregnant or breastfeeding individuals should consult with a healthcare professional before using ginseng supplements. It's important to use ginseng under the guidance of a healthcare professional and to discontinue use if any adverse effects occur.

Goldenseal:

Definition: Goldenseal, scientifically known as Hydrastis canadensis, is a perennial herb native to North America. It has a long history of use in traditional Native American medicine and later in folk medicine for its potential health benefits.

Ingredients: Goldenseal root contains various bioactive compounds, including alkaloids (such as berberine and hydrastine), flavonoids, and volatile oils. These compounds are believed to contribute to the herb's medicinal properties, including its potential as an antimicrobial, anti-inflammatory, and immune enhancer.

How to Prepare: Goldenseal is typically consumed as an herbal tea, tincture, or in supplement form (such as capsules or tablets).

To make tea, dried goldenseal root or leaves are steeped in hot water for several minutes before being strained and consumed.

Dosage: The appropriate dosage of goldenseal can vary depending on factors such as age, health status, and the specific preparation being used. It's important to follow the recommended dosage on the product label or consult with a qualified herbalist or healthcare professional for personalized guidance.

How to Use: Goldenseal tea, tincture, or supplements are typically taken orally. It's often used to support immune function, promote digestive health, and soothe inflammation.

Side Effects: Goldenseal is generally considered safe for most people when used in moderate amounts. However, some individuals may experience mild side effects such as gastrointestinal upset or allergic reactions. It may also interact with certain medications or have adverse effects in individuals with certain health conditions, such as high blood pressure or pregnancy. It's important to use goldenseal under the guidance of a healthcare professional and to discontinue use if any adverse effects occur.

Hops:

Definition: Hops, scientifically known as Humulus lupulus, is a perennial climbing vine native to Europe, Asia, and North

America. It is primarily known for its use in brewing beer but has also been used historically in traditional medicine for its potential health benefits.

Ingredients: Hops flowers contain various bioactive compounds, including bitter acids (such as humulone and lupulone), essential oils, flavonoids, and polyphenols. These compounds are believed to contribute to the herb's medicinal properties, including its potential as a sedative, relaxant, and digestive aid.

How to Prepare: Hops is typically consumed as an herbal tea, tincture, or in supplement form (such as capsules or tablets). To make tea, dried hops flowers are steeped in hot water for several minutes before being strained and consumed.

Dosage: The appropriate dosage of hops can vary depending on factors such as age, health status, and the specific preparation being used. It's important to follow the recommended dosage on the product label or consult with a qualified herbalist or healthcare professional for personalized guidance.

How to Use: Hops tea, tincture, or supplements are typically taken orally. It's often used to promote relaxation, relieve anxiety, and support sleep.

Side Effects: Hops is generally considered safe for most people when used in moderate amounts. However, some individuals may experience mild side effects such as drowsiness, gastrointestinal upset, or allergic reactions. It may also interact with certain medications or have adverse effects in individuals with certain health conditions, such as depression or hormone-sensitive conditions. It's important to use hops under the guidance of a healthcare professional and to discontinue use if any adverse effects occur.

Kelp:

Definition: Kelp refers to several species of large brown algae belonging to the Laminariales order. It is commonly found in underwater forests along rocky coastlines around the world. Kelp has been used for centuries in various cultures, particularly in East Asia, for its nutritional and medicinal properties.

Ingredients: Kelp is rich in various nutrients, including iodine, vitamins (such as vitamin K, vitamin C, and B vitamins), minerals (including calcium, magnesium, and potassium), antioxidants, and fiber. These nutrients are believed to contribute to the seaweed's potential health benefits, including its role in thyroid function, bone health, and immune support.

How to Prepare: Kelp is typically consumed dried, powdered, or in supplement form (such as capsules or tablets). It can also be used in cooking, particularly in soups, salads, and stir-fries. Kelp supplements are available in various forms, including powdered extracts, tablets, and liquid extracts.

Dosage: The appropriate dosage of kelp can vary depending on factors such as age, health status, and the specific preparation being used. It's important to follow the recommended dosage on the product label or consult with a qualified healthcare professional for personalized guidance.

How to Use: Kelp supplements are typically taken orally with water. They can be consumed as part of a daily nutritional regimen to support overall health and well-being. Kelp can also be incorporated into recipes as a flavorful and nutritious ingredient.

Side Effects: While kelp is generally considered safe for most people when consumed in moderate amounts, excessive intake of iodine-rich foods or supplements, including kelp, can lead to thyroid dysfunction or iodine toxicity. Some individuals may also be allergic to seaweed and experience allergic reactions. Pregnant or breastfeeding individuals should consult with a healthcare professional before using kelp supplements. It's important to use kelp under the guidance of a healthcare professional and to discontinue use if any adverse effects occur.

Feverfew:

Definition: Feverfew, scientifically known as Tanacetum parthenium, is a perennial herb native to Europe but also found in other parts of the world. It has a long history of use in traditional medicine, particularly in European folk medicine, for its potential health benefits.

Ingredients: Feverfew contains various bioactive compounds, including sesquiterpene lactones (such as parthenolide), flavonoids, and volatile oils. These compounds are believed to contribute to the herb's medicinal properties, including its potential as an anti-inflammatory, analgesic, and migraine prophylactic.

How to Prepare: Feverfew is typically consumed as an herbal tea, tincture, or in supplement form (such as capsules or tablets). To make tea, dried feverfew leaves and flowers are steeped in hot water for several minutes before being strained and consumed.

Dosage: The appropriate dosage of feverfew can vary depending on factors such as age, health status, and the specific preparation being used. It's important to follow the recommended dosage on the product label or consult with a qualified herbalist or healthcare professional for personalized guidance.

How to Use: Feverfew tea, tincture, or supplements are typically taken orally. It's often used to alleviate headaches, including migraines, and to support overall well-being.

Side Effects: Feverfew is generally considered safe for most people when used in moderate amounts. However, some individuals may experience mild side effects such as gastrointestinal upset or allergic reactions. It may also interact with certain medications or have adverse effects in individuals with certain health conditions, such as bleeding disorders or pregnancy. It's important to use feverfew under the guidance of a healthcare professional and to discontinue use if any adverse effects occur.

Tila:

Definition: Tila, also known as linden flower or lime blossom, refers to the flowers of the Tilia genus, primarily Tilia europaea and Tilia cordata. These trees are native to Europe, but they are also cultivated in other regions for their fragrant and medicinal flowers.

Ingredients: Tila flowers contain various bioactive compounds, including flavonoids, phenolic acids, and volatile oils. These compounds are believed to contribute to the herb's medicinal properties, including its potential as a mild sedative, anxiolytic, and anti-inflammatory agent.

How to Prepare: Tila flowers are typically prepared and consumed as an herbal tea or infusion. To make tea, dried tila flowers are steeped in hot water for several minutes before being strained and consumed.

Dosage: The appropriate dosage of tila can vary depending on factors such as age, health status, and the specific preparation being used. It's important to follow the recommended dosage on the product label or consult with a qualified herbalist or healthcare professional for personalized guidance.

How to Use: Tila tea is typically taken orally. It's often consumed in the evening as a calming bedtime beverage or during times of stress or anxiety. It's important to use tila products as directed and to discontinue use if any adverse effects occur.

Side Effects: Tila is generally considered safe for most people when used in moderate amounts. However, some individuals may experience allergic reactions or digestive upset. It may also interact with certain medications or have adverse effects in individuals with certain health conditions. It's important to use tila under the guidance of a healthcare professional and to discontinue use if any adverse effects occur.

Valerian:

Definition: Valerian, scientifically known as Valeriana officinalis, is a perennial flowering plant native to Europe and Asia. It has been used for centuries in traditional medicine for its potential calming and sedative effects.

Ingredients: Valerian root contains several bioactive compounds, including valerenic acid, valepotriates, and volatile oils. These compounds are believed to contribute to the herb's medicinal properties, including its potential as a sedative, anxiolytic, and sleep aid.

How to Prepare: Valerian root is typically prepared and consumed as an herbal tea, tincture, or capsule. To make tea, dried valerian root is steeped in hot water for several minutes before being strained and consumed. Tinctures are prepared by steeping the root in alcohol or vinegar to extract its active compounds.

Dosage: The appropriate dosage of valerian can vary depending on factors such as age, health status, and the specific preparation being used. It's important to follow the recommended dosage on the product label or consult with a qualified herbalist or healthcare professional for personalized guidance.

How to Use: Valerian tea, tincture, or capsules are typically taken orally. It's often consumed in the evening as a sleep aid or during times of stress or anxiety. It's important to use valerian products as directed and to discontinue use if any adverse effects occur.

Side Effects: Valerian is generally considered safe for most people when used in moderate amounts. However, some individuals may experience mild side effects such as drowsiness, headache, or gastrointestinal upset. It may also interact with certain medications or have adverse effects in individuals with certain health conditions. It's important to use valerian under the guidance of a healthcare professional and to discontinue use if any adverse effects occur.

THE END

9 798327 236271